"From FAT DAD
to FIT DAD in
four months!"

"From FAT DAD to FIT DAD in four months!"

Fat Loss for Dad's who don't have time and hate cardio!

Michael S. Pierron

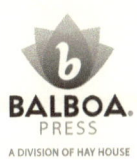

BALBOA.
PRESS

A DIVISION OF HAY HOUSE

Balboa Press books may be ordered through booksellers or by contacting:

Balboa Press
A Division of Hay House
1663 Liberty Drive
Bloomington, IN 47403
www.balboapress.com
1-(877) 407-4847

Because of the dynamic nature of the Internet, any web addresses or links contained in this book may have changed since publication and may no longer be valid. The views expressed in this work are solely those of the author and do not necessarily reflect the views of the publisher, and the publisher hereby disclaims any responsibility for them.

The author of this book does not dispense medical advice or prescribe the use of any technique as a form of treatment for physical, emotional, or medical problems without the advice of a physician, either directly or indirectly. The intent of the author is only to offer information of a general nature to help you in your quest for emotional and spiritual well-being. In the event you use any of the information in this book for yourself, which is your constitutional right, the author and the publisher assume no responsibility for your actions.

Any people depicted in stock imagery provided by Thinkstock are models, and such images are being used for illustrative purposes only.
Certain stock imagery © Thinkstock.

Printed in the United States of America

ISBN: 978-1-4525-4976-7 (sc)
ISBN: 978-1-4525-4975-0 (e)

Balboa Press rev. date: 5/23/2012

This book could have also been titled:
"Fitness Success for the Busy Baby Boomer, who is heavier than you want to be, and HATES Cardio!"

Founder of Dream BIG-
motivational speaker,
sales trainer,
comedian as the FUNNY FIT GUY and
former TALL, SKINNY and insecure kid who became a FAT DAD in his forties!

America's BIGGEST Health Challenge....our growing OBESITY epidemic!

"If you are looking for a big opportunity, seek out a BIG PROBLEM!"

Francis Pierron,

founder and president ,

P & L Construction Company, Saukville, WI (the author's Father)

CONGRATULATIONS!

You took step ONE...you or someone who cares about you bought this book.

NOW it's time...to finally get into the BEST SHAPE of YOUR LIFE!

A little background on me.

Yes, I am a BABY BOOMER...I am 48!

I'm also a son, a brother, an uncle, a SAUKVILLE SAINT (baseball player) for life, and a graduate of Grafton High School and The University of Wisconsin-WHITEWATER. My FIRST book is rated FIVE STARS on Amazon: "FIT HAPPENS at any age!"-and is a wonderful complement to the information in this E-book. You can get it direct from our family-business web site at www.drmbig.com or from Amazon.

GOOD LUCK!

"MAN must be educated to realize his greatness and to become worthy of the powers that are his."
Maria Montessori.

This year, 2011, I officially went from 298 lbs. (at The Super Bowl in late January) to 246 lbs. April 23, the day before Easter...here are my CLIFF NOTES of HOW I DID IT!

"Life is meant to be lived to the fullest!"
(Don't settle...life is too precious to waste, or to not live it FULLY)

While this utopia is nice...how attainable is it really?
I mean with marriage, the demands of a family, kids and their needs...who has TIME much less the energy to workout...well this trap was me...and every three-to-five years... I GOT FAT...again!
This last time I almost hit the magic ceiling of 300 lbs. (although my wife at the time thought I did)

The Green Bay Packers had just won the SUPER BOWL and after a 55 hour road-trip of a lifetime with our college age son Joey to watch the game...I saw PROOF that I was almost 3 BILLS!

Damn...that's enough...I'm a motivational speaker who already wrote a FIVE STAR book about motivation, fitness, and nutrition and here I go again...

Time for a NEW GOAL...and this time a BIG ONE!
To WIN a natural physique competition and QUALIFY for the masters (drug-free) Mr. Universe.

I am no different than you:

I'm a 48 year old man...1981 high school graduate.

who works for a living...

married...

two kids....one in college, one in high school,

one of 77 million baby boomers...

with gray hair...and an expanding waistline!

(I'm also tall, white and can't dance...but that's for another E-book!)

Worse yet...I'm from Wisconsin...which is good for a lot of reasons...except that our weather DOES SUCK about 6 months each year! This makes it difficult to run, walk, bike, hike...heck anything ACTIVE people do in warm weather States!

Also, being from Wisconsin, doesn't help with our diet much... our three food groups consist of "BEER, BRATS and CHESSE!"

Enough excuses...get on with the value added 44 point plan!

(why 44 points...well, it was my softball number!)

"The word 'begin' is full of energy. The best way to get something done is to begin. It's truly amazing what tasks we can accomplish if only we begin."

Clifford Warren.

What words do you see below...take your time...what do YOU see?

OPPORTUNTITYISNOWHERE.

Did you see "opportunity is NOW HERE?"
Or did you see..."opportunity is NO Where?"

First...it's our ATTITUDE we need to attack.

"People do not decide to become extraordinary. They DECIDE to accomplish extraordinary things."
Sir Edmund Hillary, the first to conquer the summit of Mount Everest.

Step ONE.
SET a specific, but BIG goal, with a DEADLINE and WRITE IT DOWN!
CLARITY accounts for probably 80% of our success and happiness.
People with "clear, concise written goals" will always accomplish far more in a shorter period of time, than people without them.
(i.e. pick a date of meaning to you in the future such as a wedding, a H.S. reunion, a cruise, a special vacation, heck even a competition... like I did)

"Where there is no vision, the people perish."
Proverbs 29:18

Step TWO.
Get your attitude in check...meaning "THIS I WILL DO!"

GREAT ATTITUDE = GREAT RESULTS
Good attitude = Good results
Fair attitude = fair results
Poor attitude = poor results.

We are NOT going to make this like a NEW YEARS RESOLUTION...one which gets blown off faster than a fake rug in a January snow storm.

This goal....we are SERIOUS about...and READY...MUST believe it's possible!

If you don't believe that it is...STOP RIGHT NOW...and start over and get YOUR ATTITUDE RIGHT!!!

Because...whether you believe it can or cannot happen...YOU ARE RIGHT! (i.e. the POWER of belief is in YOUR CONTROL....)

You can BECAUSE you think you can!
Everything is possible if you believe it's possible.
The mind tends to set limits.
What you envision you can do, you can do.
What your mind can conceive and believe,
YOU CAN ACHIEVE!
SUCCESS then is a state of mind.
Start thinking of yourself as a success.
Believe in yourself,
Know in your heart,
That you can do the job you've set out to do.
IF YOU THINK YOU CAN, YOU CAN!

Step THREE:
Take ACTION TODAY on achieving what you set out to do.
(Finish reading this E-book and order "FIT HAPPENS at any age!"-direct from us at www.drmbig.com or from Amazon.

Step FOUR:
Do something productive each day that helps you move closer to your goal!

44 PROVEN FAT-BURNING ideas...

1. Take responsibility for everything that goes into YOUR MOUTH from this moment on.

◊ More people would benefit by merely shutting their mouth and NOT EATING AS MUCH, than almost anything else I share with you.

◊ As a member of the CLEAN PLATE CLUB as a child growing up...I was PROUD to clean my plate each meal...now...I only eat until SATISFIED....NOT COMPLETELY FULL!

◊ Hello...McFly...this means you!

◊ Nutrition hint #1: Eat more meals, though smaller portions, more often. Try to eat 5-6 small meals with protein in EACH ONE!

2. Raise the bar higher than you ever thought possible. Push yourself. Get in the game, be the ball, and get MOVING!

3. DREAM BIG...and believe that getting into the best shape of your life IS POSSIBLE!

4. Move...move more...move more productively.

  ◊ Three or four weight-training workouts a week...with HIIT (high intensity interval training) cardio only! This training will keep us centered, grounded, and focused.
  ◊ Workout hint #1: Most people would benefit by "Training twice as HARD, but half as long." (i.e. raise your INTENSITY!!!!)

5. WATER. ONLY water. NO BOOZE. Alcohol is SUGAR...and for now...SUGAR is ENEMY #1! Water helps us to hydrate, detoxify and feel FULL. Plus...for dudes... it helps us to REMOVE WASTE! Hello... think big dump first thing in the morning! Also, NO POP, NO SODA, and especially NO BEER... NOTHING other than good ole H2O.for now. Don't drink any excess calories...UNLESS it's a PROTEIN shake!

6. SLEEP. 6-8 hours or whatever your body needs. Nap if at all possible, every chance you get. WHY? Your body's natural growth hormone releases when you sleep for at least 20 minutes or longer...Arnold used to call them GROWTH NAPS. If your wife was like mine, though, she thought napping made me lazy...when the opposite happened was really true and I awoke MORE REFRESHED and creative along with having much more energy.

7. GO GREEN. Eat as much GREEN STUFF as you can...broccoli, salad's (easy on the fatty dressings though) green tea, spinach etc.... Green is good! Arnold (Schwarzenegger not Palmer) once said: "If it tastes good, spit it out....if it tastes terrible...eat a lot of it." Well...he was Mr. Olympia!!!

8. Become a label reader! I'm not saying become a chick and start getting "manny's and peddy's"...but you should KNOW EXACTLY what you are eating every time. This alone will speed up your results...and help get you leaner....QUICKER.

9. Protein, protein, and more protein! As a minimum...try to eat or drink as much as one gram per pound of bodyweight...EACH and EVERY day. If you weigh 195 lbs... try to eat or drink 195 grams of protein. WHY? Protein is the only food group that CANNOT BE STORED, carbs and fat can! That's why you need to eat or drink protein every two to three hours...to help keep your metabolism high and body in balance. Protein also builds muscle, burns fat and keeps us feeling fuller longer.

◊ Don't believe me: There is a great book called "Protein POWER" written by a husband and wife Doctor team that I recommend!

10. GO NUTS! Try an ounce serving a few times a day to give your body some of the good fats it needs. Know this: "Good FAT in, bad FAT out!"

11. Don't miss a meal. It's not O.K. to skip a meal. Your body is expecting food every few hours and that's what it needs to keep your metabolism burning white hot! By skipping a meal or multiple meals you will slow your progress even more.

12. Have some protein before bed...that's right....
    you read that correct. Pass on the ice cream
    and have an ice cream flavored PROTEIN
    SHAKE, it will do your body good!

13. Mass with class. Thanks Lee Labrada! Regarding weight-training...lift as heavy as possible ALL THE TIME! Please don't believe that B.S. that "using high reps will help you get leaner, because who wants BIG ugly muscles"? NEVER has a more stupid statement been kept alive by a few million IDIOTS who don't know their head from a hole in the ground.

◊ "TRAIN for muscle...DIET for definition!" Having more muscle is your BEST FAT BURNING defense. It's been proven that by putting on one extra pound of muscle... you can eat an extra 30 -50 calories each day without gaining any weight! I know.... pretty cool! READ IT AGAIN...slower.

14. Muscle is the new skinny! LOVE that statement, and very true!

15. LIFT FIRST, CARDIO second.....ALWAYS! The idea is to try and put the most energy you have into lifting....first...when your fuel is at it's highest point and save the HIIT cardio, if you do it on the same day, for once you are into fat-burning mode. And for men it only takes us 30-35 minutes to get into fat-burning mode! Sorry ladies, for you it takes longer...45-55 minutes to get into FAT-BURNING mode.

16. HIIT is the REAL DEAL! This is the ultimate fat-burning cardio. The basic premise is to ramp up the intensity every one to two minutes and only go for 15-20 minutes HARD...to burn more total calories in less time...than those long boring steady-state cardio sessions. So even though my little brother, Bob Pierron, just completed his first IRONMAN in 12 hours, 13 minutes and 58 seconds...by swimming 2.4 miles, biking 112 miles and running a frickin marathon for 26.2 miles, I want you to do your cardio on a limited, HIGH INTENSITY proven way to burn the most fat...per minute. Safe time and GET RIPPED!

17. If you only have time for one type of training, always make it the weight-training choice... unless really sore.

18. Caffeine is fine...just no added sugar .

19. Think whey (protein) during the day and casein at night. Research proves that the body does best with protein always in your system...so keep it there.

20. GET your GLUTE ON! Glutamine that is. Supplement with five grams of glutamine before your workout and five grams after. 60% of the your muscle is glutamine, this and protein are my two MUST HALVES!

21. Training right again. GO HARD...or go HOME! INTENSITY is the key to fat loss and fat maintenance. Plus the afterburn and calories usage is off the charts for the next 24-36 hours if you have a tough "balls to the wall" workout. Don't believe me, try dead lifting or squatting for 45 minutes and see how you feel two days later?

22. ONLY EAT when your body is hungry. More often than not...you are THIRTSY not hungry. When I was younger I remember telling my Mom I'll die if I don't eat something in the next ten minutes while waiting for dinner at 4:30pm one night, she said: "drink two full glasses of water, wait five minutes and if your still hungry she'd let me eat." Never got that hungry again... IT WAS THIRST!

23. WHITE is out...GO WHOLE WHEAT!
    Arnold once said: "White bread and white
    rice is WHITE DEATH!" Try whole wheat
    pasta too...I LOVE ANGEL HAIR whole
    wheat!

24. WALK more. Park farther away from EVERYTHING....at WalMart, church, at work, at the game etc. MORE STEPS equals more fat-burning!

25. REDUCE SUGAR by half...and then half again.

26. LAUGH MORE! Go to a comedy club or rent a funny movie. Research proves that laughter is a great medicine...10-15 minutes of hearty laughter is much like a HIIT cardio session...YUCK IT UP!

27. STAY HUNGRY. Arnold starred in this movie along with Jeff Bridges and Sally Field in 1975...but the title reminds me daily...to push away from the table just a little bit hungry each time...trust me... it all adds up!

28. Jack Lalanne once said about fitness and nutrition: "EXERCISE is KING and NUTRITION is queen!" I say, treat them the same way! Both are vital to your success!

29. When trying to lose fat and maintain muscle, which is our goal...nutrition is about 80% of our battle. To get great abs.... eat chicken and broccoli and forget about all those crunches! (for now)

30. TRAIN hard...but be brief...and do NOT OVERTRAIN! Regarding each gym visit: "BE BOLD, be brief, and be gone!"

31. To get results even quicker, reduce your carb sources after 4pm each day to fiberous carbs only.

32. After your LAST MEAL of the day...brush your teeth right away. This one is so cool, I still do this every night. The mind then thinks, I'm done eating, maybe I'll read.

33. Throw your scale away, (or HIDE IT!) I do not want you weighing yourself every day. Only weigh yourself every two weeks or so to look at which way you're trending. I am ONLY concerned with your TREND line... which way are you trending.

34. PREPARE healthy food in ADVANCE. This will prevent you from "ordering a pizza" during the game when you have left-over chicken marsala in the refrigerator.

35. Have ONLY healthy snacks in the house! This prevents bingeing. I have raisons (for something sweet), peanuts, cashews and pickled herring (for something salty) and peanut butter (for something thick and goey.)

36. Form a picture in your mind of how you want to look before you start, and during your journey, to help keep you motivated. Cut out other fit people from magazines who have the body type similar to the one you aspire to and place them in a MOTIVATE ME file! Bring them to work, have them in your car, and think about the "look that you aspire too" often. This will help your motivation and energy levels.

37. UNDERSTAND, that it took years to put this weight on and "the slower it comes off, the longer it will stay off!" Your body is an incredible machine...it will help you to achieve your goal, but you need to give it a chance and let it work for you not against you.

38. "FIT HAPPENS at any age!" can help as well. In it I outline a recommended workout routine and suggest "good foods to eat." I highly encourage you read it, take notes and let the motivational right side of your brain take over!

39. SHOP for good healthy food choices. For steak, LOIN means lean, and that means Tenderloin and Sirloin are good steak choices! Yea ha!

40. Apply TNT to your new found lifestyle. TNT means training, nutrition and time. Learn proper training, match your nutrition with your goals, and allow time for it all to work.

41. INVEST in the fitness lifestyle. Understand exercise is a "two for one special." For every one hour you exercise, its proven you gain an extra two hours of quality living.

42. Think BIG muscles FIRST! Legs, back and chest are the three biggest muscles in the human body and by training them when you are fresh and full of energy, you will have the best chance to put some new muscle on and begin your fat-burning cause. Muscle is the BEST fat-burning defense you can have, it burns fat 24/7 and yes even while sleeping!

43. My goal is to live a longer, healthier and better life...by keeping this journey in proper perspective and enjoying its many benefits, you will be able to as well!

44. HAVE FAITH and be patient. It does take time, but with some effort and proper nutrition you are well on your way to a "new and improved you!"

Congratulations!

You CAN DO IT!

"It's NEVER TOO late, in fiction or in life, to REVISE!"
Nancy Thayer (author)

If you have any motivational, fitness or nutrition questions while on your weight-loss journey, feel free to email me direct at drmbig11363@yahoo.com.

Also if looking for an inspiring speaker who's style is "FUN, FAST-MOVING and has FREE STUFF" contact Mike Pierron, founder of Dream BIG at www.drmbig.com.
You can also LIKE ME on Facebook or LinkedIN.

www.ingramcontent.com/pod-product-compliance
Lightning Source LLC
Chambersburg PA
CBHW050335290526
45785CB00006B/2507